Contessa is passionate about sharing her knowledge and enthusiasm about wellness. Her many years of guiding meditation classes at workshops, corporate space and with couples have made her the face of health, youth and vitality. *12-Minute Mind Reset* is a great tool for everyone who wants a better life, deeper relationships, more sleep, happiness and love.

12-Minute Mind Reset

Contessa Hajinikitas

First published by Contessa in 2019
This edition published in 2019 by Contessa

Copyright © Contessa Hajinikitas 2019
www.wellnesswindows.com
The moral right of the author has been asserted.

All rights reserved. This publication (or any part of it) may not be reproduced or transmitted, copied, stored, distributed or otherwise made available by any person or entity (including Google, Amazon or similar organisations), in any form (electronic, digital, optical, mechanical) or by any means (photocopying, recording, scanning or otherwise) without prior written permission from the publisher.

12-Minute Mind Reset

EPUB: 9781925786576
POD: 9781925786583

Cover design by Red Tally Studios

Publishing services provided by Critical Mass
www.critmassconsulting.com

Contents

12-Minute Mind Reset	1
How This Book Will Help You To Help Yourself	3
The Wellness Immersion Scripts	6
1. Direction	15
2. Grounding	21
3. Gratefulness	26
4. Power	32
5. Prosperity	37
6. Communication Quiz	43
7. Awareness	49
8. Sleep	55
9. Confidence	59
10. Love	60
11. Zoom	61
12. 5-Minute Fix	62

12-Minute Mind Reset

Prescription for Change

How This Book Will Help You To Help Yourself

This book and the 12 wellness immersion scripts have been created to help you with your life. It is not a repeat of the many books about meditation and mindfulness that are already on the market. I don't intend to give you a lesson about the history of meditation and how you can learn to meditate in the various traditions. Nor is this book a religious piece about meditating with a particular doctrine in mind.

This book is, very simply, a way to help you to increase your concentration, become calmer and focus on what needs to be done, each and every day. In a nutshell, it is about taking control of your life.

Everyday life cannot be separated simply into 'work' and 'personal'. All parts of your life are interlinked, and should be acknowledged and celebrated – and this includes the life you may choose to have in the future. This book will give you a set of tools that you can count on every day, no matter where you are or what you are doing. These tools can make you happier and more successful; they can help you to become more aware of who you are, how you can improve yourself and how you can get along better with those around you, whether they are family, friends or colleagues.

All it takes is 12 minutes per day to change your life.

Just 12 minutes per day can improve the way you feel, shape what you believe and help you to move forward. This means no longer reacting to situations in an abrupt and uncontrollable way, but being mindful of how you respond. It means letting go of past situations and limiting beliefs that have been holding you back – in fact, letting go completely of anything that doesn't serve you. Any guilt, frustration and negativity towards the past and the present can be cleared to make way for a more purposeful today and tomorrow. This book can help you to change a pattern of running away from a situation of fear, uncertainty or boredom, or from a difficult relationship at work or home, and instead enable you to move forward of your own accord, with clarity, confidence and skill.

The wellness immersion scripts that accompany this book work in such a way that you can practise them in order throughout the week, starting on Sunday and ending on Saturday. Or you may pick and choose them to satisfy a certain requirement in your life, depending on the outcome that you wish to achieve. If you have not meditated before or it's been a long time since you did, you may like to practise the 5-Minute Fix script first, to ease you back in at a gentler pace.

Practising these scripts can improve your wellbeing in numerous ways, helping you to sleep soundly, gain confidence, take control of your emotions and become happier about life in general.

The Wellness Immersion Scripts

There are 12 wellness immersion scripts in this 12-Minute Mind Reset: one for each day of the week, designed to satisfy daily goals, plus extra scripts to evoke confidence, love, sleep, movement and a quick mind-fix.

If you'd like to complete the full-week immersion, I recommend you start on a Sunday with the Direction script as this will give you guidance and advice for the entire week.

The extra scripts can be practised on any day and at any time when particular needs are sought. For example, if you'd like to sleep more soundly, practise the Sleep immersion; if you sense that you are feeling insecure or overwhelmed, the Confidence immersion will benefit you. On the days when you feel you cannot practise a specific day's immersion or commit to the full 12 minutes, the 5-Minute Fix provides a very short script to bring you peace and the invitation to continue your longer practice when you're ready. The Zoom meditation is an active immersion for times when you'd like some movement in your practice, or simply when your energy is racing and you find it difficult to maintain a seated practice.

The scripts can either be listened to through headphones or enjoyed in a space where it's possible to relax while listening to them through speakers. By becoming familiar with the different themes, you can quickly identify which one can help you at any particular time:

1. DIRECTION
2. GROUNDING
3. GRATEFULNESS
4. POWER
5. PROSPERITY AND ABUNDANCE
6. COMMUNICATION
7. AWARENESS
8. SLEEP
9. CONFIDENCE
10. LOVE
11. ZOOM
12. 5-MINUTE FIX

1. Direction

The purpose of this immersion script is to provide you with direction for planning your week and beyond. Whether you're stuck at a crossroads with many different options to choose from, or you simply feel unable to plan the coming days, this immersion will provide clarity. It will help you to change direction from running away from what doesn't serve you, to moving towards what it is that you need.

2. Grounding

This immersion script will encourage you to feel stable and in control of your choices and decisions. Sometimes we are pulled in many different directions, perhaps serving others, and we may lose sight of what we need for our present self. This script will allow you to see things from the point of standing still and being grounded in the now.

3. Gratefulness

Practising this immersion script will help you to become very aware of what you already have, evoking feelings of gratitude, abundance, thanks and peace. Sometimes it's difficult to see what we really have – and how inside our heart we are bursting with abundance. This script helps to clarify this and encourages us to be grateful for what we already have.

4. Power

This immersion script will provide you with the way to become mentally and physically more powerful. The power will come through the process of letting go of what you have unnecessarily held on to. This is because power is depleted by holding on to something in your life that may once have been necessary, but no longer serves you. To move ahead, you must become aware of this and recognise how it has taken away your power to live and create to your full potential. The script will help to be successful, confident, happier and stronger in life, breaking free of the mundane and the predictable.

5. Prosperity and Abundance

This immersion script will help to bring abundance, health and prosperity into your life, by focusing on what is plentiful rather than highlighting what is scarce. You will be better able to gain and manifest whatever it is that you deserve and strive for, whether these wishes are physical changes or thoughts and feelings.

6. Communication

This immersion script will enable you to make NOW the time to get rid of stress, eliminate anxiety and rid yourself of negative thoughts, regrets and harmful emotions that are holding you back from being relaxed. It will help you to let go of any physical pain that has manifested in your throat and your lungs, and that may be standing in your way of clear and concise communication. Most of all, it will help you to express yourself fully and truly live your own life – a life of choice and no guilt; a life where you speak out for what is true to you.

7. Awareness

This immersion script will help you to recognise and activate your intuition and your ability to know more about yourself. This new clarity will allow you to see possibilities that you thought were impossible, allowing you to plan for the future. It will also help you to relax after the activities of the week and free you from whatever has bothered you or taken away your energy. Releasing heavy emotions from your being will enable you to enter a safe place where you can tap into your intuition and uncover what may be hidden, consciously or unconsciously – awakening you in so many ways.

8. Sleep

This immersion script will allow you to enjoy a more relaxing, peaceful and uninterrupted sleep. The deep meditation will provide you with a good night's sleep, enabling you to sleep continuously without waking up between the hours of 1 am and 3 am. The script will provide your body clock with a pattern of deep sleep.

9. Confidence

If you are lacking confidence or require validation, then this script will help you! This immersion script will allow you to reignite the confidence that you already have somewhere within you. You will be able to tackle an event or situation you feel anxious about, or successfully manage something or someone you'd like to address. The sounds and imagery will protect your self-confidence and help you conquer whatever it is that you need resolved, clarified or eliminated.

10. Love

The Love script provides the clarity required to consider and create the type of love you are aiming for.

Step by step, it addresses the love you need and the love that you want. It will help to eliminate negative feelings about love (whether conscious or unconscious) that have accumulated over your life, through your experiences with your parents, partners (past and present), and work, and free you from any burdening feelings that you've been holding on to. The immersion will make you aware and open to accept the statement: 'I deserve the love I need, I deserve the love I want.'

11. Zoom

Zoom is an active script that provides the sounds necessary to awaken the soul, the body and the mind. As you focus on the music and move to the sounds and the beat of the rhythm, it will provide you with blissful feelings and stimulate the entire being. This script can help to remedy problems with sleep, eating, body confidence and rumination.

12. 5-Minute Fix

This 5-Minute Fix is a quick immersion that will bring you feelings of relaxation and help you deal with difficult emotions that could be spoiling your day or your ability to move forward. The 5-Minute Fix can also be used by those who are new to meditation or feel that they'd like to start their practice with something shorter than the 12-minute immersions.

> **Before You Start**
>
> To make it easier, I've developed a set of quick quizzes to help you work out the best starting point for your 12-Minute Mind Reset practice. In general, these are the meanings of the answers given:
>
> Mostly A or B answers: I trust that you can start with any script you like. Focus on what you need the most today, then choose the script that will help you regain whatever it is that's important to you right now. You may learn to become more flexible in your life, understanding that it is not vital to do things perfectly every day.
>
> Mostly C answers: It would be beneficial for you to start the scripts from the beginning of the week, and, in addition to this, you may choose the subject that is most important to you today and continue with that script. You

can be negative about situations part of the time; limited beliefs can get into your way of moving forward.

Mostly D answers: Start at the beginning to get the most out of this book.

Mostly E answers: Re-read the quiz; you may have misunderstood the questions or may not have had time to fully focus on your responses.

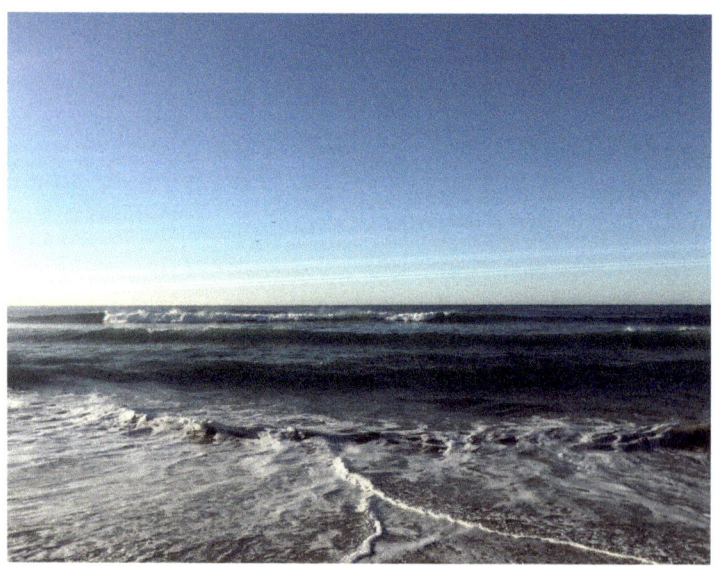

1. Direction

I recommend that you practise the Direction immersion on a Sunday – or simply whenever you need direction in your life.

Direction Quiz

Take the quiz below to understand your current state of direction and how you rate. Answer the questions honestly and count the total responses for a, b, c, d and e.

1. Do you normally start a new project when you need to, rather than procrastinating?
   a. Always
   b. Most times

c. Sometimes
   d. Never
   e. Don't know

2. Do you know which direction to take immediately, even when you're faced with more than one direction?
   a. Always
   b. Most times
   c. Sometimes
   d. Never
   e. Don't know

3. Can you follow instructions?
   a. Always
   b. Most times
   c. Sometimes
   d. Never
   e. Don't know

4. Do you usually ask questions about the task at hand to clarify what needs to be done?
   a. Always
   b. Most times
   c. Sometimes
   d. Never
   e. Don't know

5. Do you know which direction to take when given many choices?
   a. Always
   b. Most times
   c. Sometimes
   d. Never
   e. Don't know

6. Do you sigh a lot?
   a. Not usually
   b. Sometimes
   c. Most times
   d. Always
   e. Don't know

7. Do you prefer to decide on an issue with your own objectives in mind, or have someone else direct you?
   a. On my own at all times
   b. On my own most times
   c. Someone else to tell me most times
   d. Someone else to tell me at all times
   e. Don't know

8. Do you start projects at the beginning or just wherever you feel like?
   a. Always at the beginning
   b. Most of the time at the beginning

c. Sometimes at the beginning
   d. Depend on others to guide me
   e. Don't know

9. Do you have confidence in the direction you take generally in life?
   a. Always
   b. Most times
   c. Sometimes
   d. Never
   e. Don't know

10. Do you have more direction in your professional or personal issues?
    a. Both professional and personal
    b. Mainly personal issues
    c. Mainly professional issues
    d. I lack direction in both professional and personal issues
    e. Don't know

Mostly A or B answers: You are aware of the direction that you're taking, even if at times you may depend on others' objectives to set your direction. Focus on what you need the most for today and work with that. Your direction could be changed to impact you even more positively.

Mostly C answers: You tend to procrastinate when you need to decide on a direction. Don't allow any limited beliefs or negativity to prevent you from going in the direction that you need to travel in. Stay positive and continue on your chosen path. If a situation is troubling you, don't be afraid to ask questions.

Mostly D answers: You are a procrastinator and you are usually unsure about what direction to take. You often feel foggy when deciding where to go and may lack direction in both your personal and professional life. You are most successful when being guided by others, although you usually don't ask questions when taking instructions. Take your time to listen, rather than assuming you know what is required. You would be able to set goals if you were being guided, but would not feel inclined to set your own goals.

Mostly E answers: Re-read the quiz as you may have misunderstood the questions or may not have had time to fully focus on your responses.

Accentuating Your Direction Immersion

The Direction immersion can be experienced by sitting down or lying down and clicking on www.12minutemindreset.com and scroll down to 1. Direction

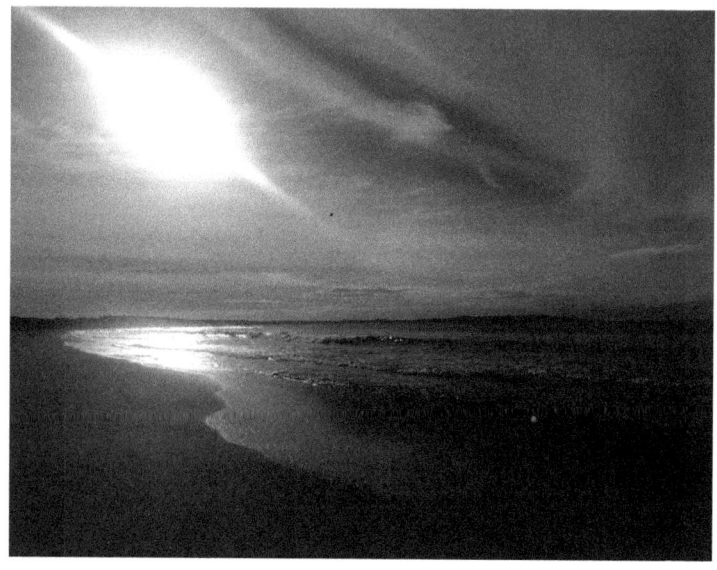

2. Grounding

It is suggested that you practise the Grounding immersion on a Monday – or whenever you need to feel more grounded.

Grounding Quiz

Take the quiz below to understand your current state of being grounded and how you rate. Answer the questions honestly and count the total responses for a, b, c, d and e.

1. How often do you feel that your head is in the clouds?
   a. Never
   b. Not often

c. Most times
   d. Always
   e. Don't know

2. Can you normally complete a task on time as planned?
   a. Always
   b. Most times
   c. Sometimes
   d. Never
   e. Don't know

3. Do you take part in any of the following activities to feel grounded?
   a. Meditation, yoga, breathing exercises
   b. Running, swimming, walking or other physical activity
   c. Reading
   d. Drinking, drugs or gambling
   e. Nothing

4. Do you suffer from headaches?
   a. No, never or seldom
   b. Yes, sometimes (once per month)
   c. Yes, a lot (every week)
   d. Always (every second day or more)
   e. Don't know

5. Do you suffer from insomnia?
   a. No, never or seldom

b. Yes, sometimes (once per month)
c. Yes, a lot (every week)
d. Always (every second day or more)
e. Don't know

6. Do you believe you are capable of anything?
    a. Always
    b. Most times
    c. Sometimes
    d. Never
    e. Don't know

7. Do you get out of control often?
    a. Never or hardly ever
    b. Sometimes
    c. Most times or often
    d. Always
    e. Don't know

8. Do you need to travel to lower levels to feel grounded?
    a. No, never
    b. Only sometimes
    c. Yes, most times
    d. Yes, always
    e. Don't know

9. Are you often unclear about your thoughts or feelings?
    a. No, never

b. Only sometimes
   c. Yes, most times
   d. Yes, always
   e. Don't know

10. Is it obvious to you when you are out of control?
    a. Yes, always
    b. Yes, most times
    c. Not often
    d. Never
    e. Don't know

Mostly A or B answers: You are very grounded and aware of the stability in your decisions. It is good to be flexible and consider whether becoming grounded in another position could improve your situation.

Mostly C answers: You are not sure what you are capable of achieving, but don't allow any limited beliefs or negativity prevent you from going to the place you need to be. Stay positive and in control; allow yourself to understand that you can be stable.

Mostly D answers: You find it difficult to be grounded and may suffer from headaches and insomnia. You often feel that you are out of control and unable to regulate your emotions and your actions. You often cannot see that you are feeling this way, which makes it more difficult to navigate.

Mostly E answers: Re-read the quiz as you may have misunderstood the questions or may not have had time to fully focus on your responses.

Accentuating Your Grounding Immersion

The Grounding immersion can be experienced by sitting down or lying down and clicking on www.12minutemindreset.com and scrolling down to 2. Grounding

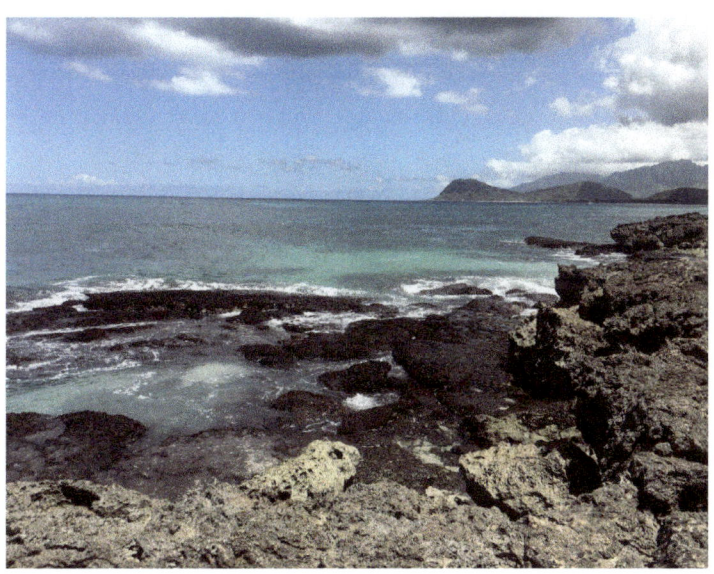

3. Gratefulness

If you are following each meditation in order from Sunday to Saturday, you will practise this Gratefulness immersion on a Tuesday – or you can choose to listen to this whenever you need to reflect upon being grateful.

Gratefulness Quiz

Take the quiz below to understand your current state of gratitude and how you rate. Answer the questions honestly and count the total responses for a, b, c, d and e.

1. Can you easily see what you have achieved on your own, or do you need to be reminded by others?
   a. I can usually or often see on my own
   b. I can sometimes see on my own

c. I usually need others to remind me
   d. I always need others to remind me
   e. Don't know

2. Do you feel grateful for what you have, or do you think about what you lack?
   a. I am usually grateful for what I already have
   b. I am mostly grateful for what I already have
   c. Usually I think about what I lack
   d. I always think about what I lack
   e. Don't know

3. Do you believe gratefulness journaling is an activity you could do in the future?
   a. Yes, I believe I can do this and it can help (or I already do this!)
   b. Yes, I believe I can do this and it may help
   c. I don't believe there is a need to do this
   d. I won't do this
   e. Don't know

4. Do you find it is easier to be grateful for your personal or your professional achievements?
   a. I am grateful for both personal and professional achievements
   b. I am grateful mostly for my professional achievements
   c. I am grateful for personal achievements

d. I usually do not feel grateful for either
   e. Don't know

5. Are you grateful for what others give to you or do for you, rather than what you do for yourself and others?
   a. I am grateful that I can help others
   b. I am grateful for both equally
   c. I am grateful when others help me
   d. I am not usually grateful
   e. Don't know

6. Do you constantly ignore what you have and focus instead on what you lack?
   a. I always focus on what I have
   b. I mostly focus on what I have
   c. I usually focus on what I lack
   d. I always focus on what I lack
   e. Don't know

7. Do others have to make you aware of what you have before you can see for yourself?
   a. I usually know for myself what I already have
   b. In general I know for myself what I have
   c. I often have to be reminded about what I have
   d. I always have to be told by others what I have
   e. Don't know

8. Do you usually tell others what they should be grateful for?
    a. I don't normally tell others what they should be grateful for; I focus on myself
    b. I sometimes remind others what they should be grateful for
    c. I often tell others what they should be grateful for
    d. I always tell others what they should be grateful for
    e. Don't know

9. How do you rate gratefulness on a scale of 0–5 (with 1 being not important and 5 being extremely important)?
    a. 5 or 4
    b. 3 or 2
    c. 1
    d. 0
    e. Don't know

10. Do you celebrate the achievement of your goals?
    a. Yes, always
    b. Yes, usually
    c. Yes, sometimes
    d. No, I am too focused on the next goal
    e. Don't know

Mostly A or B answers: You are very grateful person and you can see the riches around you, both personally and professionally. You don't usually tell others what they should be grateful for.

Mostly C answers: You usually need others to remind you of what is abundant in your life. You are mostly grateful for your personal achievements; this doesn't translate to your work achievements. You are grateful when you receive help for something. You are usually aware of what you're lacking, rather than what you have. You may tend to remind others, such as your children or work colleagues, what they should be grateful for.

Mostly D answers: Even though you are probably thankful for what you have, you tend not to acknowledge this in a conscious way. You generally focus on what you're lacking. It would be a good idea to start monitoring what exactly you do have, and that way you can give thanks for whatever you receive on a regular basis. It could help to keep a gratefulness journal.

Mostly E answers: Re-read the quiz as you may have misunderstood the questions or may not have had time to fully focus on your responses.

Accentuating Your Gratefulness Immersion

The Gratefulness immersion can be experienced by sitting down or lying down and clicking on www.12minutemindreset.com scrolling down to 3. Gratefulness

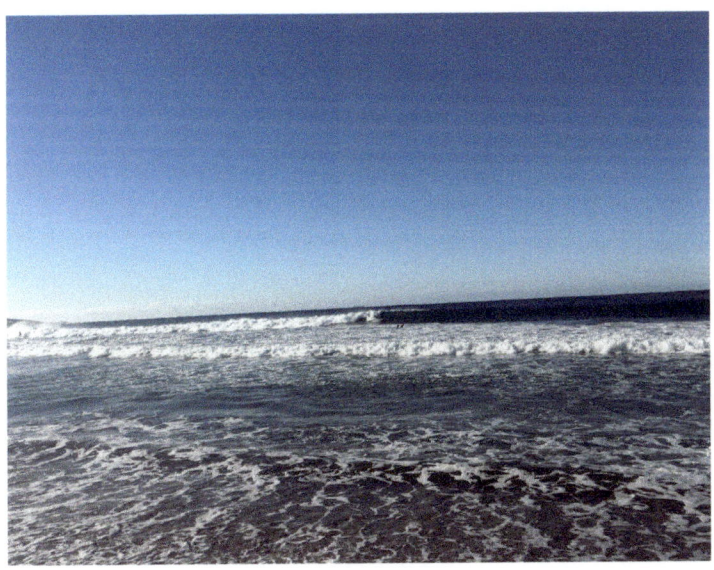

4. Power

This Power immersion will provide you with the way to become mentally and physically more powerful.

Power Quiz

Take the quiz below to understand your current state of power and how you rate. Answer the questions honestly and count the total responses for a, b, c, d and e.

1. How do you rate your power at this moment, from 0 to 5 (with 0 being powerless to 5 being extremely powerful)?
    a. 5 or 4
    b. 3 or 2
    c. 1
    d. 0
    e. Don't know

2. What do you feel takes away your power?
    a. Negative people
    b. Negative situations
    c. Unfamiliar settings
    d. Everything
    e. Don't know

3. Do you know how to increase your power every day?
    a. Usually
    b. Most times
    c. Sometimes
    d. Never
    e. Don't know

4. Is there anything you do to increase your power?
    a. Yes, I know what to do most times
    b. Yes, I know what to do sometimes
    c. Yes, I know what to do
    d. No, I don't know what to do
    e. Don't know

5. When do you feel powerless?
    a. Hardly ever
    b. Sometimes
    c. Most times
    d. All of the time
    e. Don't know

6. Do you think a powerful mind makes life easier?
   a. Yes, I believe this often
   b. Yes, I believe this sometimes
   c. I'm not sure what I believe
   d. I don't think a powerful mind makes a difference to anything
   e. Don't know

7. Do you let negative thoughts or limiting beliefs take your power away from the present?
   a. No, never
   b. Only sometimes
   c. Most of the time
   d. Always
   e. Don't know

8. Do you feel powerful in your present work?
   a. Yes, always
   b. Yes, most of the time
   c. Only sometimes
   d. Not usually
   e. Don't know

9. Do you feel powerful with making decisions at home?
   a. Yes, always
   b. Yes, most of the time
   c. Only sometimes
   d. Not usually
   e. Don't know

10. Have you ever meditated in order to restore your power?
    a. Yes, often
    b. Yes, sometimes
    c. Not usually
    d. Never
    e. Don't know

Mostly A or B answers: You rate your existing power very highly and you don't allow negative people to diminish it. You probably already meditate or undertake another activity to restore your power. You believe a powerful mind makes life easier. You don't usually let negative beliefs or limiting thoughts take away your power. You feel powerful when making both personal and professional decisions.

Mostly C answers: You may rate your existing power at a very low level (around 4 out of 10). When you are in an unfamiliar place, you feel your power is taken from you. You find it difficult to understand how to increase your daily power. Your negative thoughts and limiting beliefs will take away your power. Watch out for these.

Mostly D answers: You feel powerless. Your power is continually being taken from you by others, and by situations you don't know how to cope with. You do not know how to increase your power and you allow your limiting beliefs to become your total beliefs. You feel that you have no power around the decisions you make, and you may even believe that power is not within you.

Mostly E answers: Re-read the quiz as you may have misunderstood the questions or may not have had the time to fully focus on your responses.

Accentuating Your Power Immersion

The Power immersion can be experienced by sitting down or lying down and clicking on www.12minutemindreset.com and scrolling down to 4. Power

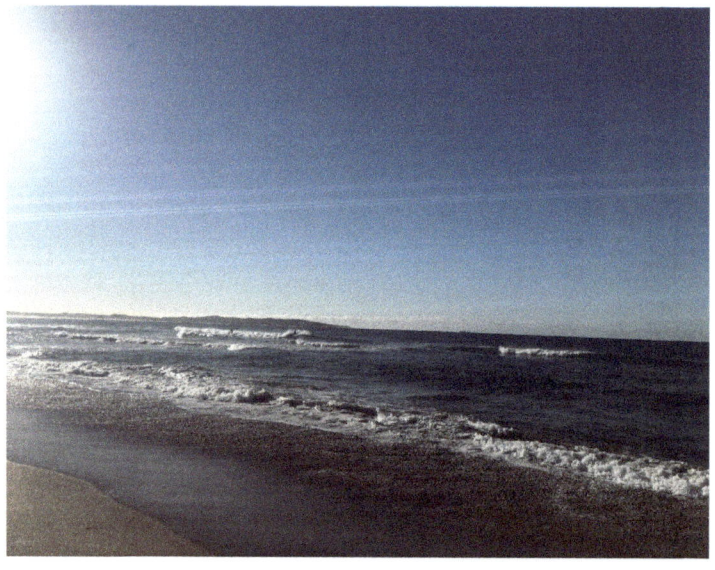

5. Prosperity

Prosperity Quiz

Take the quiz below to understand your current state of prosperity and how you rate. Answer the questions honestly and count the total responses for a, b, c, d and e.

1. How do you rate your prosperity at this moment? Rate this from 0 to 5, with 0 being not all prosperous to 5 being extremely prosperous.
    a. 5 or 4
    b. 3
    c. 2 or 1
    d. 0
    e. Don't know

2. What is your top issue of prosperity?
   a. Health/family
   b. Money
   c. Work
   d. Pleasure
   e. Don't know

3. Do you want to increase your prosperity?
   a. Yes, a lot
   b. Yes, a moderate amount
   c. Yes, a little
   d. Not really
   e. Don't know

4. Is there anything you can do that will increase your prosperity?
   a. Yes, I always have ways
   b. Yes, I have a few ways
   c. I am usually not sure
   d. I don't care
   e. Don't know

5. Do you think prosperity is something that you can gain or something you're born with?
   a. I can gain much more prosperity if I wish
   b. I can gain a little more prosperity if I wish
   c. I'm not sure if I can gain prosperity

d. Prosperity is something we are born with
   e. Don't know

6. Is it necessary to work hard to achieve prosperity?
   a. It depends on what you're doing
   b. Working hard is important
   c. Working hard could work
   d. Hard work is overrated
   e. Don't know

7. Do you think abundance is a limited resource?
   a. There is a plentiful supply for everyone and it's everywhere
   b. There is a plentiful supply if you know where to look
   c. There is abundance in some areas
   d. Abundance is a limited resource
   e. Don't know

8. Do you ever discuss the abundance in your life?
   a. Yes, I discuss abundance a lot
   b. Yes, I discuss abundance some of the time
   c. No, I don't think I need to discuss this
   d. What is abundance?
   e. Don't know

9. Can you see your life becoming more prosperous in the future?

a. Yes, always
   b. Yes, most of the time
   c. Yes, sometimes
   d. Never
   e. Don't know

10. Do you have any beliefs or values that you believe are keeping you from greater prosperity?
    a. No, I don't think I have anything that's really keeping me from reaching greater prosperity
    b. I have a few beliefs and values that are keeping me from reaching greater prosperity
    c. I have many beliefs that are keeping me from reaching a greater prosperity
    d. My beliefs and values will always stop me from becoming prosperous
    e. Don't know

Mostly A and B answers: You feel prosperous and rate your present level at around 7–8+ out of 10. Your top issues of prosperity are probably health, family and money. You know your prosperity isn't limited and you are capable of finding ways to increase your prosperity that are not just related to hard work. You discuss prosperity in your daily life and know that prosperity is not a limited resource, believing there is enough for everyone.

Mostly C answers: You feel your prosperity is rated at 3–4 out of 10. You believe prosperity comes from work or the ability of others. You are not sure how to increase your prosperity apart from working hard. You don't usually discuss the abundance of your life with others. Your beliefs may be limiting your ability to increase the prosperity in your life. Be careful that negative thoughts don't determine what you can truly achieve in your life.

Mostly D answers: You believe that prosperity is something that we are born with and that it is difficult to increase our prosperity in life. You aren't really sure if there is a need to discuss your prosperity with anyone. In the past you haven't been able to work hard to increase your prosperity.

Mostly E answers: Re-read the quiz as you may have misunderstood the questions or may not have had the time to fully focus on your responses.

Accentuating Your Prosperity Immersion

The Prosperity immersion can be experienced by sitting down or lying down and clicking on www.12minutemindreset.com and scrolling down to 5. Prosperity and Abundance

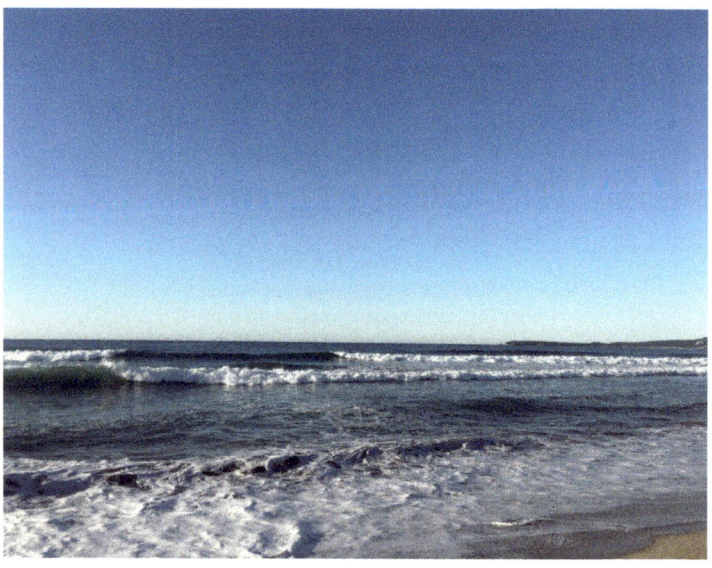

6. Communication Quiz

Take the quiz below to understand how you communicate. Answer the questions honestly and count the total responses for a, b, c, d and e.

1. In conversations are you normally the one who talks or the one who listens?
   a. I usually communicate with balanced talking and listening
   b. Most of the time I communicate with balanced talking and listening
   c. I talk most of the time and don't listen much
   d. I talk all of the time or I am totally silent
   e. Don't know

2. When meeting new people do you usually remember names a week afterwards?
    a. Yes, I usually remember most people's names
    b. Yes, I remember people's names if I think I will see them again
    c. Yes, I remember the names of people who can serve me
    d. I forget most names
    e. Don't know

3. Do you fear speaking in front of an audience? Rate on a scale of 0–5 with 0 being not fearful at all and 5 being extremely fearful.
    a. 0 or 1
    b. 2
    c. 3 or 4
    d. 5
    e. Don't know

4. Do you believe that your communication is a combination of both your conscious and subconscious minds?
    a. Yes, I believe this most times
    b. Yes, I believe this sometimes
    c. There could be a link, but I'm not sure
    d. I don't believe this
    e. Don't know

5. Do you read books (e-books included)?
   a. Yes, I always have a book with me
   b. Yes, I have a book with me most of the time
   c. Yes, I have a book with me sometimes
   d. I don't generally read much
   e. Don't know

6. How often do you talk to your family or significant other about what is important to them?
   a. We talk every day
   b. We talk most days
   c. We only talk some of the time
   d. We don't really talk much and/or I feel there is some distance
   e. Don't know

7. At work, do you use your power to talk down to others to get what you need?
   a. No, never
   b. Yes, sometimes
   c. Yes, most of the time
   d. Yes, always – this is my right
   e. Don't know

8. Are you a confident in your ability to communicate?
   a. Yes, usually or always
   b. Yes, most times
   c. Yes, sometimes

d. Not really
   e. Don't know

9. Do you think you can convince others when you speak?
   a. Yes, I believe I'm convincing most or all of the time
   b. Yes, I believe I'm convincing a lot of the time
   c. Yes, I believe I'm convincing sometimes
   d. I don't think I can convince others
   e. Don't know

10. Do you think you can be persuaded to change your mind or behaviour based on listening to someone's speech or reasons?
    a. Yes, I believe I can change my mind and I have an open mind most of the time
    b. Yes, I believe I can change my mind and I have an open mind sometimes
    c. I believe in what I believe – there's no need to change anything
    d. I am unsure either way
    e. Don't know

Mostly A or B answers: In conversations, you usually demonstrate a balance of talking and listening. You usually remember others' names long after meeting them. You feel confident about public speaking and are mostly prepared for your presentations. You understand that what you don't say is just as important as what you do say. You enjoy learning and often read or listen to personal development material. You talk to your partner and family about what issues are important to you and them. Your mind is open to change and you are willing to learn from others' understanding of a topic.

Mostly C answers: You are probably the one talking most of the time, rather than the one who is listening. You generally don't have a good memory for people's names, but can usually recall if you think you will see the person again or especially if the person can be of future assistance. You may be a confident speaker one to one but find it difficult in giving a presentation to a large group of people. You don't tend to talk to you partner or family about what is important to them. You may be prone to talking down to others such as children, work colleagues and your spouse. You are not inclined to change your existing viewpoint in response to listening to a presentation.

Mostly D answers: In your 'conversations', you are either silent all the time or unable to hear anything other than your own voice! You are not very good at remembering other people's names and would find it difficult – if not impossible – to make a presentation in front of a large audience. You may not be talking much to the important people in your life and you may be avoiding these conversations by watching television or using electronic devices.

Mostly E answers: Re-read the quiz as you may have misunderstood the questions or may not have had the time to fully focus on your responses.

Accentuating Your Communication Immersion

The Communication immersion can be experienced by sitting down or lying down and clicking on www.12minutemindreset.com and scrolling down to 6. Communication

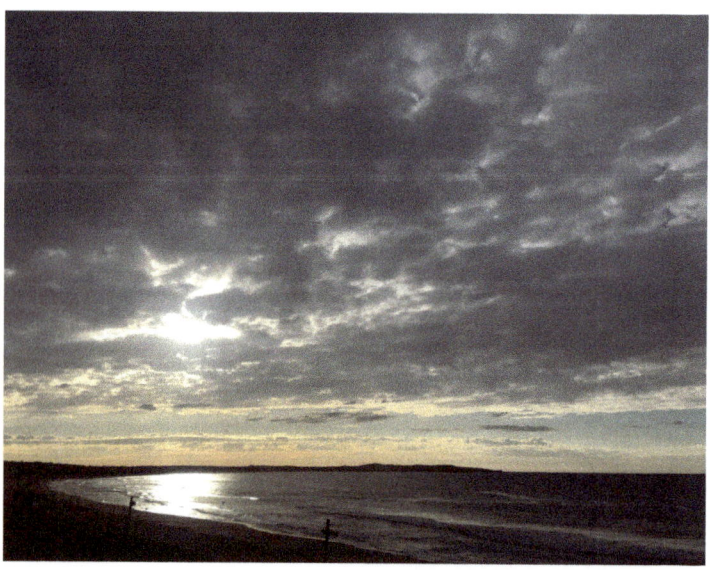

7. Awareness

Awareness Quiz

Take the quiz below to understand your current state of awareness and how you rate. Answer the questions honestly and count the total responses for a, b, c, d and e.

1. How aware are you of your feelings?
   a. I am very aware of my feelings most or all of the time
   b. I am aware of my feelings sometimes
   c. I have some awareness of my feelings when I focus
   d. I don't really feel too aware of my feelings most of the time
   e. Don't know

2. How aware are you of others' feelings?
   a. I am very aware of others' feelings most of the time
   b. I am aware of others' feelings when I have known them for a long time
   c. I am aware of others' feelings when it suits me
   d. I'm not really aware of how others feel
   e. Don't know

3. How aware are you of where a conversation is going?
   a. I am very aware most of the time
   b. I am very aware sometimes
   c. I have moments of awareness
   d. I'm not very aware
   e. Don't know

4. Are you aware of how to change the subject of a conversation if it is going off track?
   a. Yes, I am very aware of how to do this
   b. Yes, I am aware of how to do this
   c. Sometimes I am aware of how to do this
   d. I'm not very aware
   e. Don't know

5. Do you know what you plan to do in the next 5 years?
   a. Yes, I have a clear plan and I will adjust it to suit changes in life
   b. Yes, I have a basic plan

c. I have a plan but I haven't committed to it
   d. I don't make future plans
   e. Don't know

6. Are you aware of your surroundings?
   a. Yes, I am very aware and can describe my surroundings in detail
   b. Yes, I am somewhat aware
   c. I am aware at that moment, but cannot recall anything later
   d. I don't take too much notice of my surroundings
   e. Don't know

7. Can you remember people's names after you've met them?
   a. Yes, usually or always
   b. Yes, most of the time
   c. Yes, sometimes
   d. Not really
   e. Don't know

8. Do you have goals to achieve for the week?
   a. Yes, I have my goals and a strategy on how to achieve them
   b. Yes, I have my goals
   c. Yes, I have some ideas about what I want to do
   d. I don't really have any goals – life will happen anyway
   e. Don't know

9. Are you aware of your breath when you close your eyes and focus?
   a. Yes, I'm aware of this most of the time and find it easy to do
   b. Yes, I'm aware of this sometimes and find it easy to do
   c. Yes, I'm aware but I find this difficult to achieve
   d. I'm not aware of my breath
   e. Don't know

10. Do you listen to or read any self-development material regularly i.e. at least 4 times per week?
    a. Yes, every week
    b. Yes, most weeks
    c. Yes, most months
    d. Sometimes
    e. Never or don't know

Mostly A or B answers: You are very aware of your own feelings and others' feelings most of the time. Even if you cannot relate to the other person's experience you can empathize with the situation. You usually have clarity about the subject of your conversation and can identify when a conversation is going off the subject. You have goals, and strategies to achieve those goals for the short term (1 week) and for the longer term (5 years). You are usually aware of your surroundings and know they can influence your situation. You are aware of your breath when you close your eyes. You probably have a regular self-development ritual that you follow.

Mostly C answers: When you focus, you have some awareness of your feelings. You are aware of other people's feelings sometimes, although usually this corresponds with whether the other person can help you or not. When a conversation is going off track, you find it difficult to focus and come back to the topic. You have a vague plan about what you will do for the next 5 years but are unsure if you can fully commit to the plan. Your weekly goals are clear and you have some idea of how to achieve these. Sometimes you remember people's names after meeting them but this is not common. You are not usually aware of your breath when you focus. You would use self-development material if it was made available to you and you did not have to invest much into it.

Mostly D answers: From the answers you have given, it seems that you are not aware of how you and others are feeling most of the time. When you are having a conversation, you often find yourself not sticking to the subject at hand. Once this happens, you find it difficult to return to the topic. You are not aware of your short- or long-terms goals and allow life to cruise past. It would be very helpful to commence reading or listening to self-development material.

Mostly E answers: Re-read the quiz as you may have misunderstood the questions or may not have had the time to fully focus on your responses.

Accentuating Your Awareness Immersion

The Awareness immersion can be experienced by sitting down or lying down and clicking on www.12minutemindreset.com and scrolling down to 7. Awareness

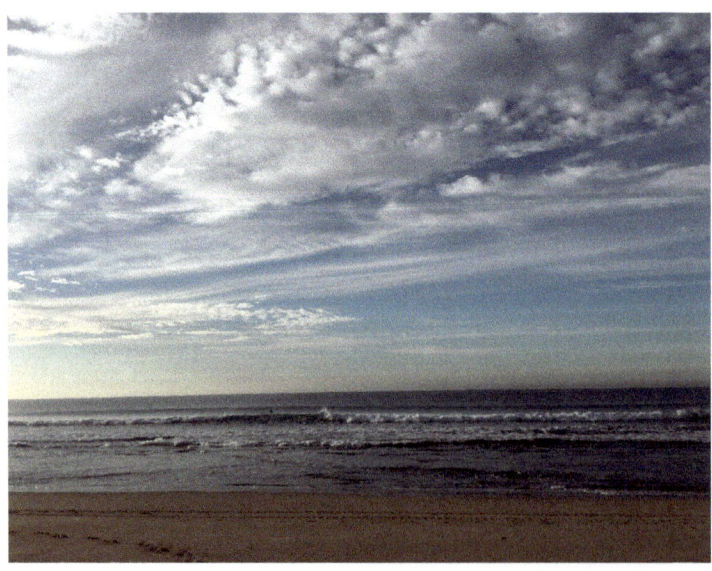

8. Sleep

Accentuating Your Sleep Immersion

Take the quiz below to understand your current state of sleep and how you rate. Answer the questions honestly and count the total responses for a, b, c, d and e.

1. Do you sleep soon after you go to bed?
    a. Yes, every night
    b. Yes, most nights
    c. No, I don't get to sleep most nights
    d. I can never get to sleep
    e. Don't know

2. Do you wake up during the night?
    a. No, never

b. Hardly ever
   c. Sometimes
   d. Most nights or always
   e. Don't know

3. Do you eat or drink anything 90 minutes before bedtime?
   a. No, never
   b. Hardly ever
   c. Sometimes
   d. Most nights or always
   e. Don't know

4. How many hours do you sleep soundly every night?
   a. 6–8 hours
   b. 5–6
   c. 4–5
   d. Fewer than 4
   e. Don't know

5. Do you use your computer or electronic device or watch television an hour prior to sleeping?
   a. No, never
   b. Hardly ever
   c. Sometimes
   d. Most nights or always
   e. Don't know

6. Do you take any health supplements on a regular basis?
   a. Yes, every day
   b. Yes, most days
   c. Sometimes, but not regularly
   d. Never or hardly ever
   e. Don't know

7. Have you experienced any of the following major events in the past 18 months?
   a. Relationship issue such as divorce or death
   b. Change of living arrangements, such as moving into a new house or relocating overseas
   c. Having child/children
   d. Other event
   e. Don't know

8. Do you suffer from any of the following: heart disease, diabetes, high blood pressure, muscle/joint pain, sore back?
   a. None
   b. 1 or 2
   c. 3 or 4
   d. All
   e. Don't know

9. Do you do any of the following: smoke cigarettes 3–5 times per week; consume more than 7

alcoholic drinks per week; smoke marijuana at least once per week, or other drugs most days?
a. None
b. 1 or 2
c. 3
d. All of the above
e. Don't know

10. Is it completely dark in your bedroom?
a. Yes, always
b. Yes, most nights
c. Only sometimes
d. My room is usually bright
e. Don't know

The Sleep immersion can be experienced by sitting down or lying down and clicking on www.12minutemindreset.com and scrolling down to 8. Sleep

9. Confidence

Accentuating Your Confidence Immersion

The Confidence immersion can be experienced by sitting down or lying down and clicking on www.12minutemindreset.com and scrolling down to 9. Confidence

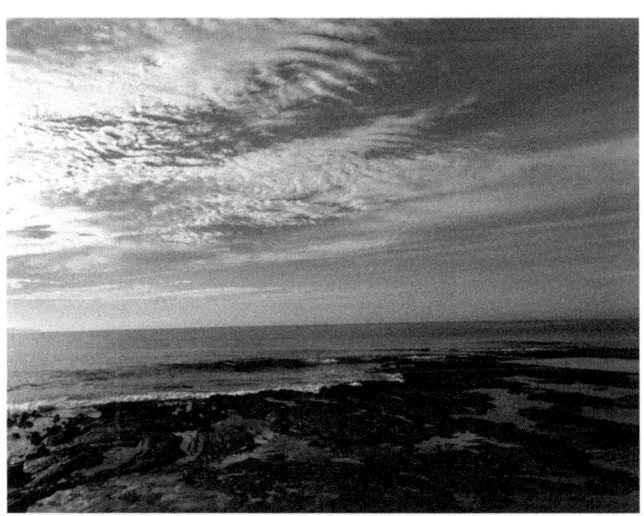

10. Love

Accentuating your Love Immersion

The Love immersion can be experienced by sitting down or lying down and clicking on www.12minutemindreset.com and scrolling down to 10. Love

11. Zoom

Accentuating Your Zoom Immersion

The Zoom immersion can be experienced by sitting down or lying down and clicking on www.12minutemindreset.com and scrolling down to 11. Zoom

12. 5-Minute Fix

Accentuating Your 5-Minute Fix Immersion

The 5-Minute Fix immersion can be experienced by sitting down or lying down and clicking on www.12minutmindreset.com and scrolling down to 12. 5 Minute Fix

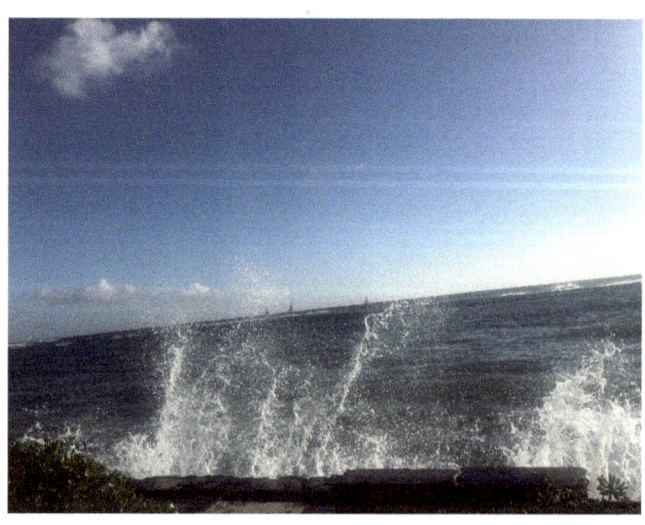